# DIABETES DIET RECIPES COOKBOOK

Lose Weight, Boost Your Metabolism and Stay Healthy, Including Simple and Delicious Recipes.

## Lory Ason

**Copyright © 2021** Lory Ason

# Table of content

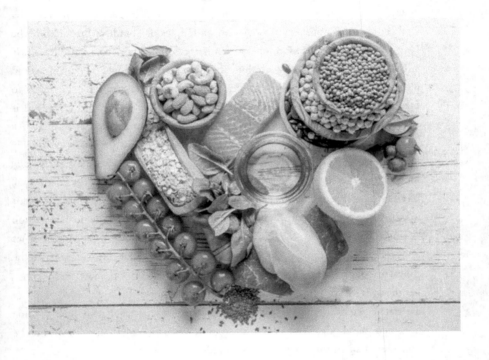

# Introduction to Diabetes

What is Diabetes?
Diabetes Mellitus is not a single hereditary disease but a heterogeneous group of diseases, all of which ultimately lead to an elevation of glucose in the blood (hyperglycaemia) and loss of glucose in the urine as hyperglycaemia increases.

It is also characterised by the three "polys" and inability to reabsorb water, resulting in increased urine production (polyurea) excessive thirst (polydipsia) and excessive eating (polyphagia).

## Type 1 Diabetes

Occurs abruptly, characterised by an absolute deficiency of insulin due to a marked decline in the number of insulin producing beta cells (perhaps caused by the auto immune destruction of beta cells) even though target cells contain insulin receptors.

Type 1 diabetes is also known as insulin dependant diabetes and juvenile onset diabetes, as it most commonly develops in people under 20 years old though it persists through life, and requires periodic insulin injections to treat it.
Although type 1 diabetes appears to have certain genes which make them more susceptible, some triggering factor is required e.g. viral infection, shock etc.

**Type 2 Diabetes**

It most often occurs in people who are over forty and overweight hence another name "maturity onset diabetes". Clinical symptoms are mild, and high glucose levels in the blood can usually be controlled by diet, exercise, and/or with anti diabetic drugs.

Some type II diabetes have sufficient amounts of insulin in the blood, but they have defects in the molecular machinery that mediates the action of insulin on its target cells, cells can become less sensitive to insulin because they have fewer insulin receptors.

Type II diabetes is therefore called non-insulin dependant diabetes. 90% of all cases are type II.

The Pancreas

The pancreas can be classified as both an endocrine and exocrine gland. Thus it is referred to as a heterocrine gland, but we will only be looking at its endocrine functions here. The pancreas is a flattened organ located posterior and slightly inferior to the stomach. The adult pancreas consists of a head, body and tail. The pancreas contains approx. one million clusters of inlets of langerhans. Three kinds of cells are found in these clusters.

## Glucagon

This hormones principle physiological activity is to increase the blood glucose level. It does this by accelerating the conversion of glycogen into glucose (glycogenesis) which the liver then releases into the bloodstream.

Secretion of glucagon is directly controlled by the level of blood sugar via a negative feedback system. When the blood sugar level falls below a certain level chemical sensors in the alpha cells of the inlets stimulate the cells to secrete glucagon. Once the blood sugar level has risen cells are no longer stimulated, and production slackens. Glucagon secretion is inhibited by GHIH (samastostatin).

## Insulin

Insulin is produced by the inlet Beta cells, and acts to lower blood sugar levels. It does this by accelerating the transport of glucose from the blood into cells (especially muscle). Glucose entry into cells depends on the presence of insulin receptors on the surface of the target cells. It also accelerates the conversion of glucose into glycogen (glycogenesis).

Insulin also decreases gluconeogenesis and glycogenolysis, stimulates the conversion of glucose and of other nutrients into fatty acids (lipogenesis), and helps stimulate protein synthesis.

Insulin secretion is based on a negative feedback system related to blood sugar levels.

Other hormones do affect insulin production eg. samatostatin inhibits selection.

As insulin production of the body usually depends upon the amount of carbohydrate intake and also the amount of carbohydrate used in exercise etc. Insulin intake must be constantly balanced against them.

# Classic Omelet and Greens

Try this for a dinner-worthy omelet
Simple yet delicious, this omelet is elegant enough for dinner, and easy enough for breakfast or brunch. Serve with a side of lemony greens to make the meal complete!

## Ingredients

3 tbsp. olive oil, divided
1 yellow onion, finely chopped
8 large eggs
Kosher salt
2 tbsp. unsalted butter
1 oz. Parmesan, finely grated
2 tbsp. fresh lemon juice
3 oz. baby spinach

## Directions

Heat 1 tablespoon oil in large nonstick skillet on medium. Add onion and sauté until tender, about 6 minutes. Transfer to a small bowl.
In a large bowl, whisk together eggs, 1 tablespoon water and 1/2 teaspoon salt.
Return skillet to medium and add butter. Add eggs and cook, stirring constantly with rubber spatula, until eggs are partially set. Turn heat to low and cover pan tightly, cooking until eggs are just set, 4 to 5 minutes. Top with Parmesan and cooked onion; fold in half.
In a medium bowl, whisk together lemon juice and remaining 2 tablespoons olive oil. Toss spinach with vinaigrette and serve

with omelet.

NUTRITIONAL INFORMATION (per serving): About 330 calories, 27.5 g fat (9.5 g saturated), 16 g protein, 575 mg sodium, 6 g carbohydrates, 1 g fiber

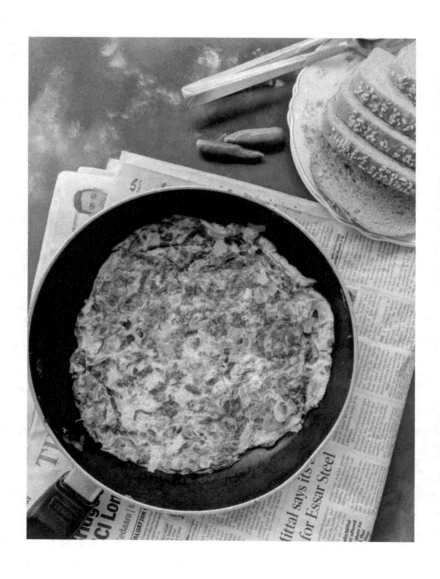

# Berry Yogurt Bowl

Fill up before you start your day with a bowl of this berry yogurt. If you're looking to spice things up, swap the berries for apple or pear slices.

## Ingredients

3/4 c. plain 2% Greek yogurt
1 tbsp. Chopped mint
2 1/2 tbsp. chopped walnuts
1/2 c. Citrus and Mint Berries

## Directions

Spoon the yogurt into a bowl. Top with Citrus and Mint Berries, mint and walnuts.
Eat fresh or keep chilled.

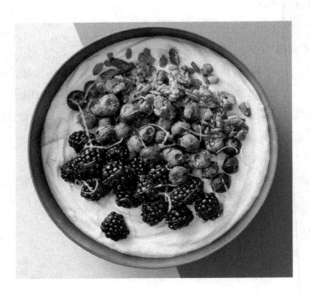

# Avocado Toast Recipe

This Avocado Toast is my go to breakfast and is so incredibly easy to make! It's so delicious, made with tasty ingredients and takes only 10 minutes!

## Ingredients

2 slices bread I love Dave's Killer Bread because it's lower in carb that regular breads and higher in healthy fats
½ medium avocado (mine weighed 9.7oz with the large pit still inside 6.1pz with the pit removed and avocado still in skins
⅛ teaspoon Sea salt
1/8 teaspoon Black pepper
Juice of 1/2 lime
A few slices of pickled onions recipe here
sprinkle of Red pepper flakes
optional: a shake of everything bagel seasoning

## Instructions

Toast your bread until golden brown.
While your bread is toasting, scoop out your avocado from the skin and place it in a bowl. Squeeze in the lime, and sprinkle in the sea salt and black pepper. Using a fork, mash it until it's to the texture you prefer.
Spread the avocado on the toasts evenly.
Sprinkle/put on the rest of the topics and enjoy!

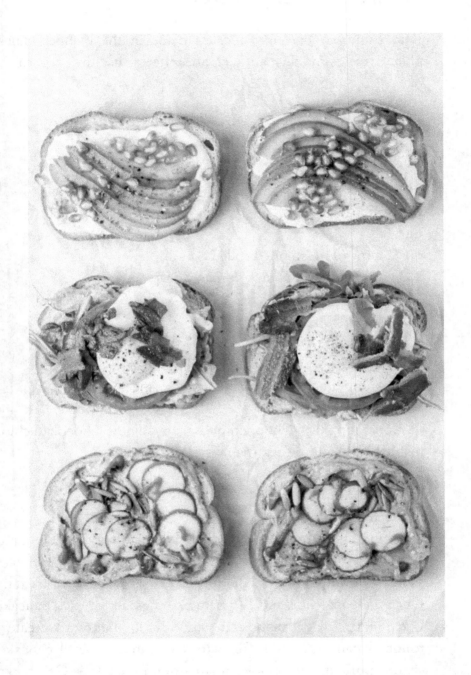

# Pumpkin Protein pancakes

Easy Pumpkin Protein Pancakes made in the blender! These gluten free pumpkin pancakes are an easy, healthy start to the day.

## Equipment
Blender
Large skillet or griddle

## Ingredients

1 1/2 cups old-fashioned rolled oats
2/3 cup pumpkin puree (sub mashed ripe banana)
1/2 cup full-fat cottage cheese (I use Good Culture brand)
2 large eggs
2 Tbsp. maple syrup
2 tsp. baking powder
1 tsp. pumpkin pie spice (sub apple pie spice)
1/4 tsp. salt
Optional toppings: Chopped pecans or walnuts, chocolate chips, maple butter, nut butter, maple syrup.
Instructions

## Direction
Combine all ingredients in a high power blender; blend until mostly smooth. Let batter sit in the blender while you preheat a skillet (or griddle) over medium heat. Grease with oil or butter.
Once the pan is hot, add 1/3 batter to the pan for each pancake. Use the back of a spoon to smooth out batter to create a rounded pancake. Cook for 2 to 4 minutes, or until pancakes slightly puff up and bubbles form around the edges. Gently flip,

and cook another 1 to 2 minutes, or until golden brown on the underside. (Note: if the pancakes start browning too quickly, reduce heat to medium-low to prevent burning.) Serve warm with toppings of choice.

Notes

To Store: Place leftover pancakes in an airtight storage container and refrigerate for up to 4 days.

To Reheat: Gently rewarm pancakes in the microwave until hot. Alternatively, you can also reheat them on a baking sheet in the oven at 350°F until warmed through, or in a toaster oven.

To Freeze: First, allow your pancakes to fully cool. Once cooled, place a piece of parchment or wax paper in between each pancake and stack them on top of one another. Transfer to a freezer-safe gallon ziptop bag, and freeze for up to 3 months. When ready to eat, reheat pancakes directly from frozen as instructed.

**Nutrition**

Serving: 3pancakes | Calories: 295kcal | Carbohydrates: 41g | Protein: 16g | Fat: 7g | Saturated Fat: 2g | Sodium: 400mg | Fiber: 5g | Sugar: 12g

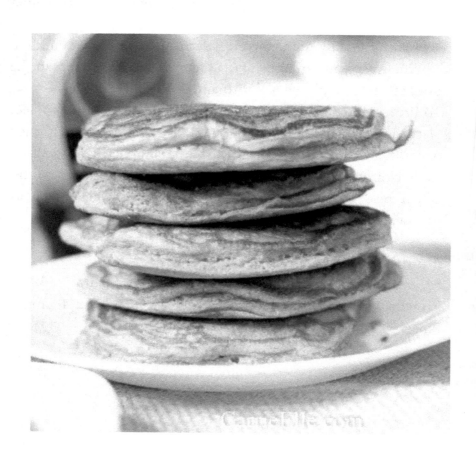

# Best-Ever Granola

One easy granola, five different ways.

## Ingredients

1/2 c. olive oil or extra virgin coconut oil (melted)
3/4 c. pure maple syrup
2 tbsp. turbinado sugar (we used Sugar in the Raw)
1 tsp. kosher salt
3 c. old-fashioned rolled oats
1 c. unsweetened coconut flakes
3/4 c. raw sunflower seeds
3/4 c. raw pumpkin seeds

## Directions

Best-Ever Granola
Heat oven to 300°F. Line large rimmed baking sheet with parchment paper. In large bowl, combine oil, maple syrup, sugar, and salt. Add oats, coconut and sunflower and pumpkin seeds and stir to evenly coat.
Spread mixture onto prepared baking sheet and bake, stirring every 15 min., until granola is light golden brown and dry, 45 to 55 minutes. Let cool completely.
For Ginger-Pecan Granola: Omit pumpkin seeds and reduce sunflower seeds to 1/2 cup. Add 1 1/2 cups pecans (roughly chopped). Bake granola per recipe instructions, tossing with 1 1/2 tablespoon grated fresh ginger (from one 2-inch piece) when it comes out of oven.
For Cumin-Thyme Granola: Omit coconut. Add 2 tablespoon each cumin seeds and fresh thyme leaves and 1 teaspoon

ground cinnamon to bowl along with oil and maple syrup.

For Spicy Sesame-Tamari Granola: Omit sugar, salt, and sunflower seeds. Use only 1/2 cup coconut and increase pumpkin seeds to 1 cup. Stir in 1/2 cup tamari with oil and add 1/2 cup sesame seeds and heaping 1/2 tsp cayenne along with oats.

For Coriander-Almond Granola: Omit sugar, coconut, and pumpkin seeds. Add 1/4 cup coriander seeds (lightly crushed) and 1 1/2 cups sliced almonds along with oats.

For Sweet and Spicy Granola: Omit coconut and increase pumpkin and sunflower seeds to 1 1/2 cups each. Bake granola per recipe instructions, tossing with 1 1/2 teaspoon ground cinnamon and 1 teaspoon chipotle chile powder when it comes out of oven.

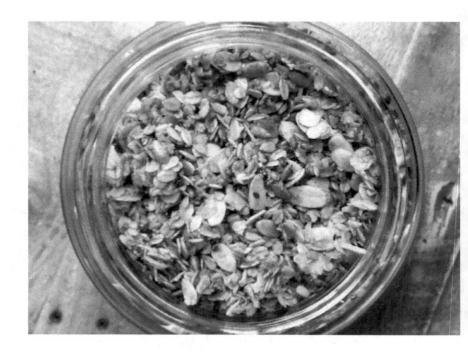

# Gruyère, Bacon, and Spinach Scrambled Eggs

A few add-ins make this breakfast staple feel fancy
A touch of Dijon mustard, salty bacon, melty cheese, and a handful of greens seriously upgrades scrambled eggs, without too much effort!

## Ingredients

8 large eggs
1 tsp. Dijon mustard
Kosher salt and pepper
1 tbsp. olive oil or unsalted butter
2 slices thick-cut bacon, cooked and broken into pieces
2 c. spinach, torn
2 oz. Gruyère cheese, shredded

## Directions

In a large bowl, whisk together eggs, Dijon mustard, 1 tablespoon water and 1/2 teaspoon each salt and pepper.
Heat oil or butter in 10-inch nonstick skillet on medium. Add eggs and cook, stirring with rubber spatula every few seconds, to desired doneness, 2 to 3 minutes for medium-soft eggs. Fold in bacon, spinach, and Gruyère cheese.

# Fruity Yogurt Parfait

Start your day with a colorful, healthy dish.

## Ingredients

1 c. frozen mixed berries
c. non-fat Greek yogurt
1 tbsp. flaxseed
tsp. vanilla extract
1/2 kiwi
1/4 c. blueberries
3 tbsp. Kind Healthy Grains Fruit & Nut Clusters

## Directions

In food processor or blender, pulse frozen berries, yogurt, flaxseed, and vanilla extract until smooth.
Transfer yogurt mixture to bowl; top with kiwi, blueberries, and Fruit & Nut Clusters.

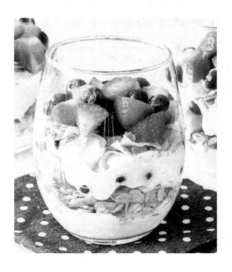

# Chilled Overnight Chia

Wake up to this dreamy, creamy breakfast that "cooks" itself overnight.

## Ingredients

Milk & Honey
2 c. old-fashioned oats
4 tbsp. chia seeds
4 tbsp. honey
milk or unsweetened plant-based milk
Blueberry-Coconut
2 c. old-fashioned oats
4 tbsp. chia seeds
4 tbsp. honey
3 c. light coconut milk
1 tsp. lemon zest
fresh blueberries
Brownie Batter
2 c. old-fashioned oats
4 tbsp. chia seeds
4 tbsp. honey
milk or unsweetened plant-based milk
4 tbsp. Unsweetened cocoa powder
4 tbsp. chocolate-hazelnut spread
chopped toasted hazelnuts
PB&J
2 c. old-fashioned oats
4 tbsp. chia seeds
4 tbsp. honey

milk or unsweetened plant-based milk
4 tbsp. peanut butter
4 tbsp. Strawberry jam
Sliced strawberries

## Directions

Milk & Honey: To each of four 16-ounce jars, add 1/2 cup oats, 1 tablespoon chia seeds, 1 tablespoon honey, and 2/3 milk. Cover; shake to combine. Refrigerate.

Blueberry-Coconut: To each of four 16-ounce jars, add 1/2 cup oats, 1 tablespoon chia seeds, 1 tablespoon honey, and 3/4 cup coconut milk. Cover; shake to combine and refrigerate. To serve, stir 1/4 teaspoon lemon zest into each jar and top with blueberries.

Brownie Batter: To each of four 16-ounce jars, add 1/2 cup oats, 1 tablespoon chia seeds, 1 tablespoon honey, 2/3 milk, 1 tablespoon and cocoa powder. Cover; shake to combine and refrigerate. After soaking, stir 1 tablespoon chocolate-hazelnut spread into each jar; top with hazelnuts.

PB&J: To each of four 16-ounce jars, add 1/2 cup oats, 1 tablespoon chia seeds, 1 tablespoon honey, and 2/3 milk. Cover; shake to combine and refrigerate. After soaking, stir in 1 tablespoon peanut butter and top each jar with 1 tablespoon strawberry jam and strawberries.

PER SERVING (MILK & HONEY) 365 CAL, 12 G PRO, 57 G CAR, 12 G FAT (4 G SAT), 8 G FIBER, 70 MG SODIUM

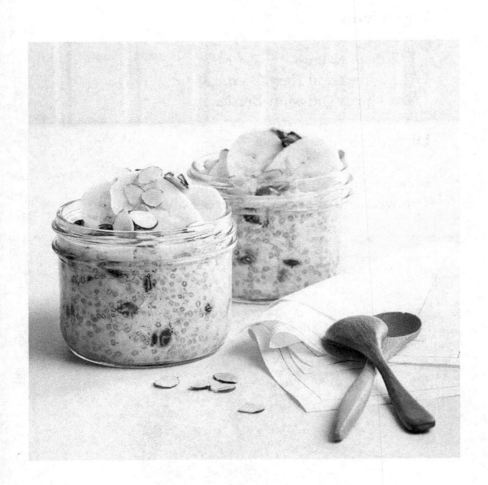

## Berry Oatmeal

This is the protein-packed (and fruity!) breakfast you'll look forward to eating.

### Ingredients

1 1/2 tbsp. walnuts
1/2 c. Quick and Easy Oatmeal
1/2 c. Citrus and Mint Berries

### Directions

Reheat Quick and Easy Oatmeal.
Top with Citrus and Mint Berries and walnuts

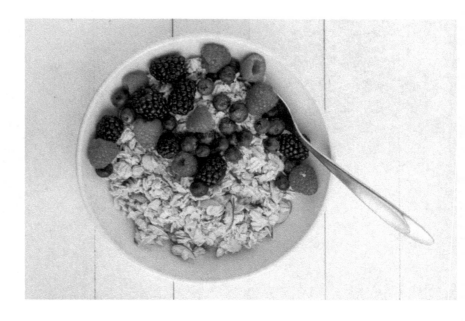

# Summer Smoothies

Sip on summer's fruitiest flavors with these four easy-to-make recipes.

## Ingredients
Mango Madness
1 c. orange juice
1/2 c. coconut yogurt
1 1/2 c. frozen mango
1 medium carrot, coarsely grated
Strawberry Fields
1/2 c. coconut water
1/2 c. coconut yogurt
1 c. strawberries
1/2 c. frozen peaches
Green Goddess
1/2 c. unsweetened almond milk
1/2 c. honey yogurt
2 bananas, cut into pieces and frozen
3 c. baby spinach
Razzle-Dazzle
1/2 c. low-fat milk
1/2 c. nonfat Greek yogurt
2 c. frozen raspberries
2 bananas, peeled and cut into pieces

## Directions
In blender, puree the ingredients until smooth.
To make smoothie bowl: Make Razzle-Dazzle Smoothie and transfer to bowls. Top with kiwi slices, coconut flakes, and raspberries.

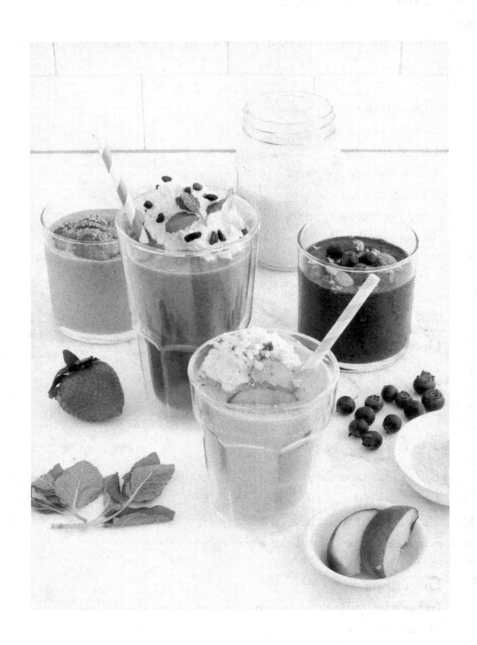

# Steak and Eggs

**Ingredients** - Allergies: SF, GF, DF, NF

- 1/4 lb boneless beef steak or pork tenderloin
- 1/4 tsp ground black pepper
- 1/4 tsp sea salt (optional)
- 1 tsp coconut oil
- 1/4 onion, diced
- 1/2 red bell pepper, diced
- 1 handful spinach or arugula
- 1 egg Instructions

## Directions

Season sliced steak or pork tenderloin with sea salt and black pepper. Heat a sauté pan over high heat. Add 1 tsp coconut oil, onions, and meat when pan is hot, and sauté until steak is slightly cooked. Add spinach and red bell pepper, and cook until steak is done to your liking. Meanwhile, heat a small fry pan over medium heat. Add remaining coconut oil, and fry two eggs. Top steak with a fried egg to serve.

## Precooked beans

Again, some recipes require that you cook some beans (butter beans, red kidney, garbanzo) in advance. Cooking beans takes around 3 hours and it can be done in advance or every few weeks and the rest get frozen. Soak beans for 24 hours before cooking them. After the first boil, throw the water, add new water and continue cooking. Some beans or lentils can be sprouted for few days before cooking and that helps people with stomach problems.

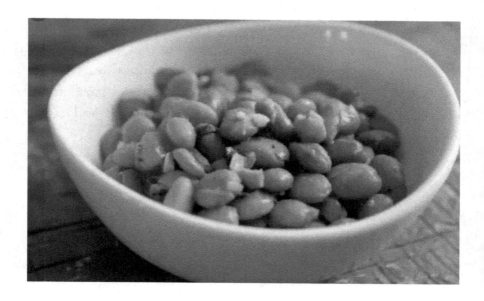

# Tomato paste

Some recipes (chili) require tomato paste. I usually prepare 20 or so liters at once (when tomato is in season, which is usually September) and freeze it.

## Ingredients

5 lbs. chopped plump tomatoes
1/4 cup extra-virgin olive oil or avocado oil plus 2 tbsp.
salt, to taste

## Instructions - Allergies: SF, GF, DF, EF, V, NF

Heat 1/4 cup of the oil in a skillet over medium heat. Add tomatoes. Season with salt. Bring to a boil. Cook, stirring, until very soft, about 8 minutes.
Pass the tomatoes through the finest plate of a food mill. Push as much of the pulp through the sieve as possible and leave the seeds behind.
Bring it to boil, lower it and then boil uncovered, so the liquid will thicken (approx. 30-40 minutes). That will give you homemade tomato juice. You get tomato paste if you boil for 60 minutes, it gets thick like store bought ketchup.
Store sealed in an airtight container in the refrigerator for up to one month, or freeze, for up to 6 months.

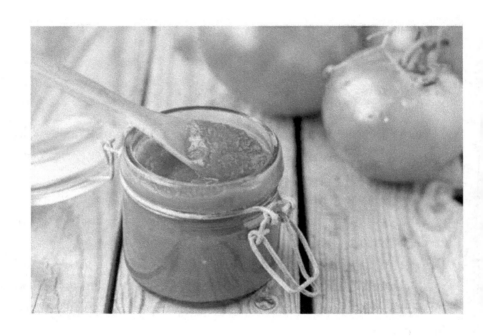

# Curry Paste

This should not be prepared in advance, but there are several curry recipes that are using curry paste and I decided to take the curry paste recipe out and have it separately. So, when you see that the recipe is using curry paste, please go to this part of the book and prepare it from scratch. Don't use processed curry pastes or curry powder; make it every time from scratch. Keep the spices in original form (seeds, pods), ground them just before making the curry paste. You can dry heat in the skillet cloves, cardamom, cumin and coriander and then crush them coarsely with mortar and pestle.

## Ingredients

2 onions, minced
2 cloves garlic, minced
2 teaspoons fresh ginger root, finely chopped
6 whole cloves
2 cardamom pods
2 (2 inch) pieces cinnamon sticks, crushed
1 tsp. ground cumin
1 tsp. ground coriander
1 tsp. salt
1 tsp. ground cayenne pepper
1 tsp. ground turmeric

**Instructions** - Allergies: SF, GF, DF, EF, V, NF

Heat oil in a frying pan over medium heat and fry onions until transparent. Stir in garlic, cumin, ginger, cloves, cinnamon, coriander, salt, cayenne, and turmeric. Cook for 1 minute over medium heat, stirring constantly. At this point other curry ingredients should be added.

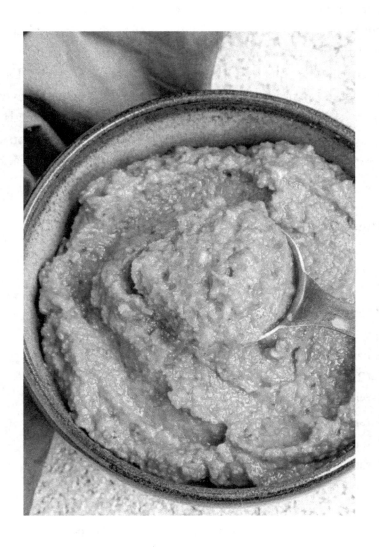

# Cocoa Oatmeal

**Ingredients** - Allergies: SF, GF, DF, NF

1/2 cup dry oats
1 cup water
A pinch tsp. salt
1/2 tsp. ground vanilla bean
1 tbsp. cocoa powder
1 tbsp. lucuma powder
3 tbsp. ground flax seeds meal
a dash of cinnamon
2 egg whites

## Instructions

In a saucepan over high heat, place the oats and salt. Cover with water. Bring to a boil and cook for 3-5 minutes, stirring occasionally.
Keep adding 1/2 cup water if necessary as the mixture thickens.
In a separate bowl, whisk 4 tbsp. water into the 1 tbsp. cocoa powder to form a smooth sauce. Add the vanilla to the pan and stir.
Turn the heat down to low. Add the egg whites and whisk immediately. Add the flax meal, and cinnamon. Stir to combine.
Remove from heat, add lucuma powder and serve immediately.
Topping suggestions: sliced strawberries, blueberries or few almonds.

# Apple Oatmeal

**Ingredients -** Allergies: SF, GF, DF, EF, V, NF

1/2 grated apple
1/2 cup dry oats
1 cups water
Dash of cinnamon
1 tsp. lucuma powder

## Instructions

Cook the oats with the water for 3-5 minutes.
Add grated apple and cinnamon. Stir in the lucuma powder.

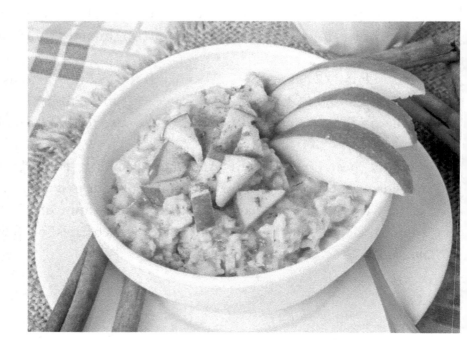

# Coconut Pomegranate Oatmeal

**Ingredients** - Allergies: SF, GF, DF, EF, V, NF
1/2 cup dry oats
1/3 cup coconut milk
1 cups water
2 tbs. shredded unsweetened coconut
1 tbs. flax seeds meal
1 tbs. lucuma powder
4 tbs. pomegranate
seeds

## Instructions

Cook oats with the coconut milk, water, and salt.
Stir in the coconut, lucuma powder and flaxseed meal. Sprinkle
with extra coconut and pomegranate seeds.

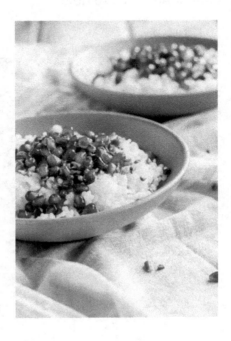

# Egg Muffins

**Ingredients** - Allergies: SF, GF, DF, NF

Serving: 4 muffins
4 eggs
1/2 cup diced green bell pepper
1/2 cup diced onion
1/2 cup spinach
1/4 tsp. salt
1/8 tsp. ground black pepper
2 tbsp. water

## Instructions

Heat the oven to 350 degrees F. Oil 4 muffin cups. Beat eggs together. Mix in bell pepper, spinach, onion, salt, black pepper, and water. Pour the mixture into muffin cups. Bake in the oven until muffins are done in the middle.

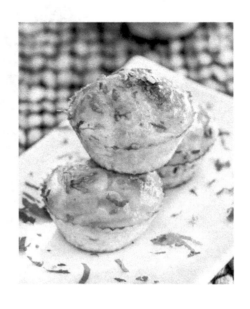

# Smoked Salmon Scrambled Eggs

**Ingredients** - Allergies: SF, GF, DF, NF

1 tsp coconut oil
2 eggs
1 Tbs water
2 oz smoked salmon, sliced
1/4 avocado
ground black pepper, to taste
2 chives, minced (or use 1 green onion, thinly sliced)

## Instructions

Heat a skillet over medium heat. Add coconut oil to pan when hot. Meanwhile, scramble eggs. Add eggs to the hot skillet, along with smoked salmon. Stirring continuously, cook eggs until soft and fluffy. Remove from heat. Top with avocado, black pepper, and chives to serve.

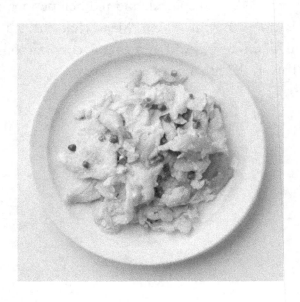

# Steak and Eggs

## Ingredients - Allergies: SF, GF, DF, NF

1/4 lb boneless beef steak or pork tenderloin
1/4 tsp ground black pepper
1/4 tsp sea salt (optional)
1 tsp coconut oil
1/4 onion, diced
1/2 red bell pepper, diced
1 handful spinach or arugula
1 egg

## Instructions

Season sliced steak or pork tenderloin with sea salt and black pepper. Heat a sauté pan over high heat. Add 1 tsp coconut oil, onions, and meat when pan is hot, and sauté until steak is slightly cooked. Add spinach and red bell pepper, and cook until steak is done to your liking. Meanwhile, heat a small fry pan over medium heat. Add remaining coconut oil, and fry two eggs. Top steak with a fried egg to serve.

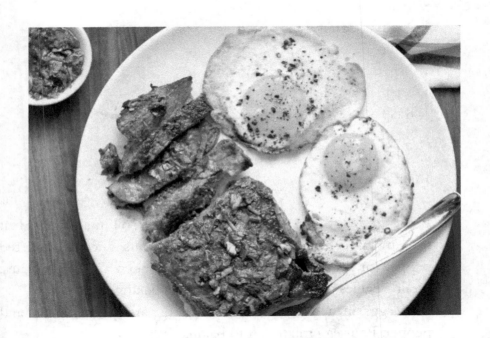

# Egg Bake

**Ingredients** - Allergies: SF, GF, DF, NF

1/2 cup chopped red peppers or spinach
1/4 cup zucchini
1/2 tbsp. coconut oil
1/4 cup sliced green onions
2 eggs
1/4 cup coconut milk
1/8 cup almond flour
1 tbsp. minced fresh parsley
1/4 tsp. dried basil
1/8 tsp. salt
1/8 tsp. ground black pepper

## Instructions

Preheat oven to 350 degrees F. Put coconut oil in a skillet. Heat it to medium heat. Add mushrooms, onions, zucchini and red pepper (or spinach) until vegetables are tender, about 5 minutes. Drain veggies and spread them over the baking dish.

Beat eggs in a bowl with milk, flour, parsley, basil, salt, and pepper. Pour egg mixture into baking dish.

Bake in preheated oven until the center is set (approx. 35 to 40 minutes).

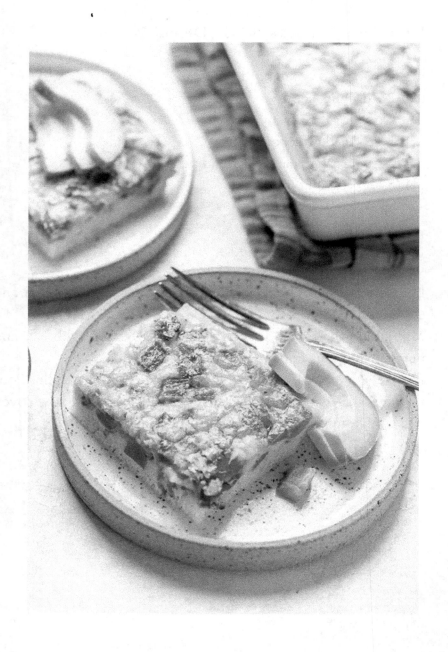

# Frittata

## Ingredients - Allergies: SF, GF, DF, NF

1 tbsp. olive oil or avocado oil
1/2 Zucchini, sliced
1/4 cup torn fresh spinach
1 tbsp. sliced green onions
1/4 tsp. crushed garlic, salt and pepper to taste
1/8 cup coconut milk
2 eggs

## Instructions

Heat olive oil in a skillet over medium heat. Add zucchini and cook until tender.

Mix in spinach, green onions, and garlic. Season with salt and pepper. Continue cooking until spinach is wilted.

In a separate bowl, beat together eggs and coconut milk. Pour into the skillet over the vegetables. Reduce heat to low, cover, and cook until eggs are firm (5 to 7 minutes).

# Superfoods Naan Pancakes Crepes

## Ingredients - Allergies: SF, GF, DF, EF, V

1/2 cup almond flour
1/2 cup Tapioca Flour
1 cup Coconut Milk
Salt
Coconut oil

## Instructions

Mix all the ingredients together.
Heat a pan over medium heat and pour batter to desired thickness. Once the batter looks firm, flip it over to cook the other side.
If you want this to be a dessert crepe or pancake, then omit the salt. You can add minced garlic or ginger in the batter if you want, or some spices.

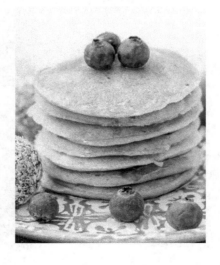

# Zucchini Pancakes

**Ingredients** - Allergies: SF, GF, DF

1 small zucchini
1 tbsp. chopped onion
2 beaten eggs
3 tbsp. almond flour
1/2 tsp. salt
1/2 tsp. ground black pepper
Coconut oil

**Instructions**

Heat the oven to 300 degrees F. Grate the zucchini into a bowl and stir in the onion and eggs. Stir in 6 tbsp. of the flour, salt, and pepper.
Heat a large sauté pan over medium heat and add coconut oil in the pan. When the oil is hot, lower the heat to medium-low and add batter into the pan. Cook the pancakes about 2 minutes on each side, until browned. Place the pancakes in the oven.

# Greek Salad

**Allergies**: SF, GF, EF, NF

1 head romaine lettuce
1/2 lb. plump tomatoes
3 oz. Greek or black olives, sliced
2 oz. sliced radishes
4 oz. low-fat feta or goat cheese
2 oz. anchovies (optional)

**Dressing:**
2 oz. olive oil or avocado oil
2 oz. fresh lemon juice
1/2 tsp. dried oregano
1/4 tsp. black pepper
1/4 tsp. salt
2 cloves garlic, minced

**Directions**
Wash and cut lettuce into pieces. Slice tomatoes in quarters. Combine olives, lettuce, tomatoes, and radishes in large bowl. Mix dressing ingredients together and toss with vegetables. Pour out into a shallow serving bowl. Crumble feta/goat cheese over all, and arrange anchovy fillets on top (if desired).

# Strawberry Spinach Salad

Ingredients - Allergies: SF, GF, DF, EF, V

1 tbsp. black sesame seeds
1 tbsp. poppy seeds
1/4 cup olive oil or cumin oil
1/8 cup lemon juice
1/8 tsp. paprika
1/2 bag fresh spinach - chopped, washed and dried
1 cup strawberries, sliced
1/4 cup toasted slivered almonds

## Instructions

Whisk together the sesame seeds, olive oil, poppy seeds,
paprika, lemon juice and onion. Refrigerate.
In a large bowl, combine the spinach, strawberries and almonds.
Pour dressing over salad. Toss and refrigerate 15 minutes before
serving.

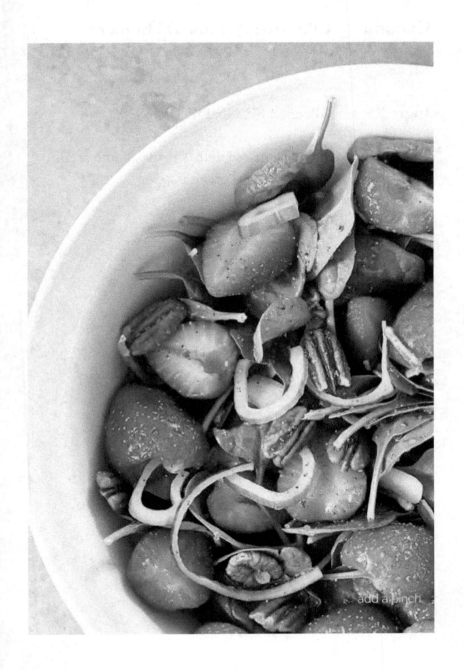

# Cucumber, Cilantro, Quinoa Tabbouleh

Serves 2

**Ingredients -** Allergies: SF, GF, DF, EF, NF, V

1/2 cup cooked quinoa mixed with 1 tbsp. sesame seeds
1/2 cup chopped tomato and green pepper
1 cup chopped cucumber
1/2 cup chopped cilantro Dressing:
1 tbsp. olive oil or avocado oil
1 tbsp. fresh lemon juice
pinch of black pepper
pinch of sea salt

**Instructions**

Mix all ingredients.

# Almond, Quinoa, Red Peppers & Arugula Salad

Serves 2

**Ingredients** - Allergies: SF, GF, DF, EF, NF, V

1/2 cup cooked quinoa mixed with 1 tbsp. pumpkin seeds
1/2 cup chopped almonds
1 cup chopped arugula
1/2 cup sliced red peppers Dressing:
1 tbsp. olive oil or cumin oil
1 tbsp. fresh lemon juice
pinch of black pepper
pinch of sea salt

**Instructions**

Mix all ingredients.

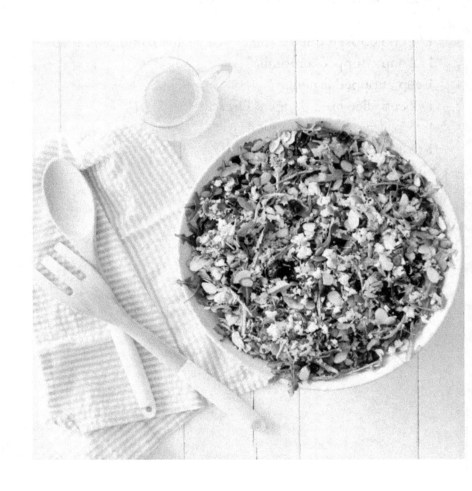

# Asparagus, Quinoa & Red Peppers Salad

Serves 2

**Ingredients** - Allergies: SF, GF, DF, EF, NF, V

1/2 cup cooked quinoa mixed with 1 tbsp. sunflower seeds
1 cup sliced red peppers
1 cup grilled asparagus
Garnish with lime and parsley
Dressing:
1 tbsp. olive oil or avocado oil
1 tbsp. fresh lemon juice
pinch of black pepper
pinch of sea salt

**Instructions**

Mix all ingredients.

# Chickpeas, Quinoa, Cucumber & Tomato Salad

Serves 2

**Ingredients** - Allergies: SF, GF, DF, EF, NF, V

1/2 cup cooked quinoa mixed with 1 tbsp. sesame seeds
1/2 cup cooked chickpeas
1 cup chopped cucumber and green onions
1/2 cup chopped tomato Dressing:
1 tbsp. olive oil or avocado oil
1 tbsp. fresh lemon juice
pinch of black pepper
pinch of sea salt

**Instructions**

Mix all ingredients.

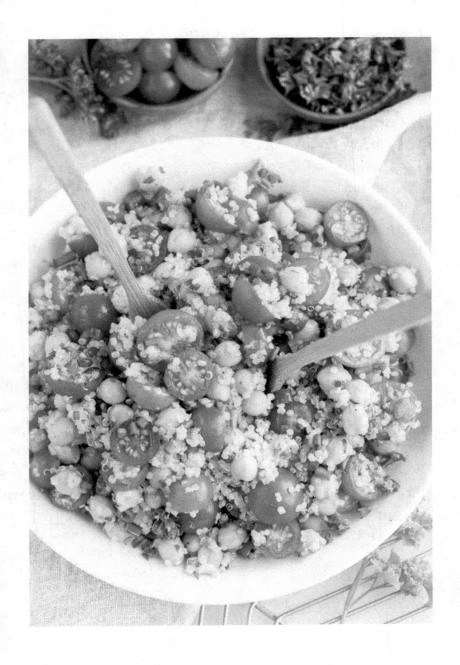

# Quinoa Salad

**Ingredients** - Allergies: SF, GF, EF

For the salad
1/2 cup cooked quinoa
1/2 cup frozen green peas
1/4 cup low-fat feta cheese
4 oz. pork, cubed
1/8 cup freshly chopped basil and cilantro
1/8 cup almonds, pulsed in a food processor until crushed for the dressing
1/8 cup lemon juice (1 juicy lemon)
1/8 cup olive oil or cumin oil
1/8 tsp. salt (more to taste)

## Instructions

Bring a pot of water to boil and then lower the heat. Add the peas and cook covered until bright green. In the meantime, brown pork in a skillet. Toss the quinoa with the pork, peas, feta, herbs, and almonds.

Puree all the dressing ingredients in the food processor. Toss the dressing with the salad ingredients. Season generously with salt and pepper. Serve tossed with fresh baby spinach.

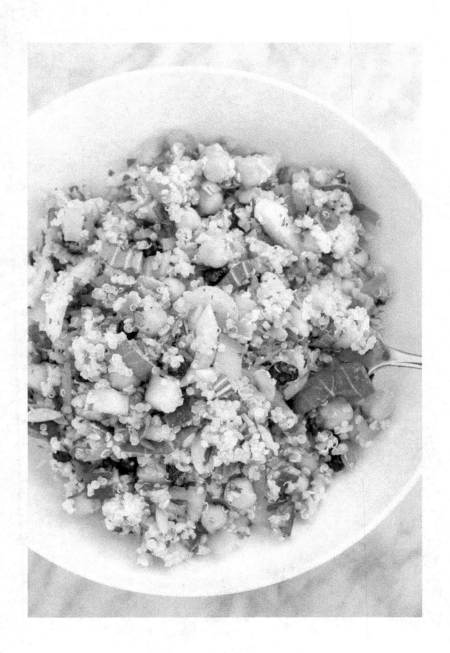

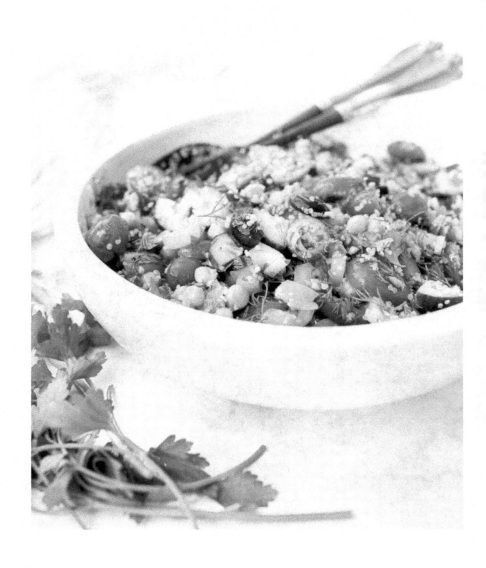

# Cauliflower & Eggs Salad

**Ingredients** - Allergies: SF, GF, NF

1 cup chopped Cauliflower
2 hardboiled eggs - chopped,
2 oz. shredded cheddar cheese, low-fat
1/2 red onion, celery,
1 dill pickles,
1 tbsp. yellow mustard.

## Instructions

Mix all ingredients.

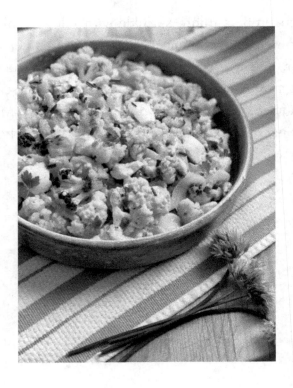

# Greek Cucumber Salad

**Ingredients** - Allergies: SF, GF, EF, NF

2 cucumbers, sliced
1 teaspoon salt
2 tbsp. lemon juice
1/4 tsp. paprika
1/4 tsp. white pepper
1/2 clove garlic, minced
2 fresh green onions, diced
1 cup thick Greek Yogurt
1/4 tsp. paprika

**Instructions**

Slice cucumbers thinly, sprinkle with salt and mix. Set aside for one hour. Mix lemon juice, water, garlic, paprika and white pepper, and set aside. Squeeze liquid from cucumber slices a few at a time, and place slices in the bowl. Discard liquid. Add lemon juice mixture, green onions, and yogurt. Mix and sprinkle additional paprika or dill over top. Chill for 1-2 hours.

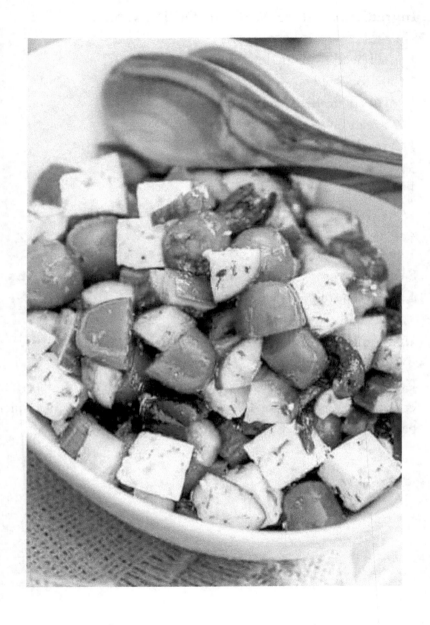

# Mediterranean Salad

**Ingredients** - Allergies: SF, GF, DF, EF, V, NF

1 small head romaine lettuce, torn
1 tomato, diced
1 small cucumber, sliced
1/2 green bell pepper, sliced
1/2 small onion, cut into rings
3 radishes, thinly sliced
1/4 cup flat leaf parsley, chopped
1/4 cup olive oil or avocado oil
2 tbsp. lemon juice
1 garlic clove, minced
Salt & pepper
1 tsp. fresh mint, minced

**Instructions**

Combine lettuce, tomatoes, cucumber, pepper, onion, radishes
& parsley in a salad bowl. Whisk together olive oil, lemon juice,
garlic, salt, pepper & mint. Pour over salad & toss to coat.

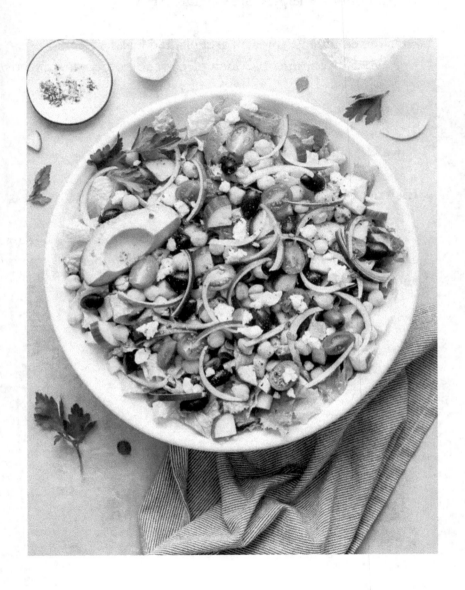

# Pomegranate Avocado salad

**Ingredients** - Allergies: SF, GF, DF, EF, V

cups mixed greens, spinach, arugula, red leaf lettuce
ripe avocado, cut into 1/2-inch pieces cup pomegranate seeds
1/2 cup pecan
1/2 cup blackberries
1/2 cup cherry tomatoes
Olive oil, salt, lemon juice

## Instructions

Combine greens, pecan, cut avocado, tomatoes, pomegranates and blackberries in a salad bowl. Whisk together salt, olive oil and lemon juice and pour over salad.

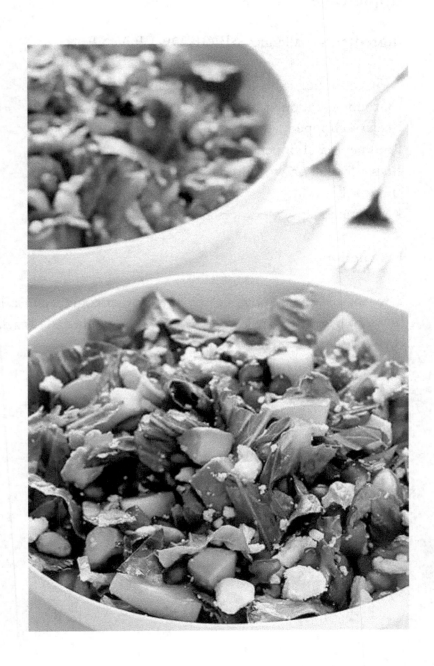

# Apple Coleslaw

**Ingredients** - Allergies: SF, GF, DF, EF, V, NF

2 cups chopped cabbage (various color)
1 tart apple chopped
1 celery, chopped
1 red pepper chopped
4 tsp. olive oil or avocado oil
juice of 1 lemon
1 Tbs. lucuma powder (optional dash sea salt)

## Instructions

Toss the cabbage, apple, celery, and pepper together in a large bowl. In a smaller bowl, whisk remaining ingredients. Drizzle over coleslaw and toss to coat.

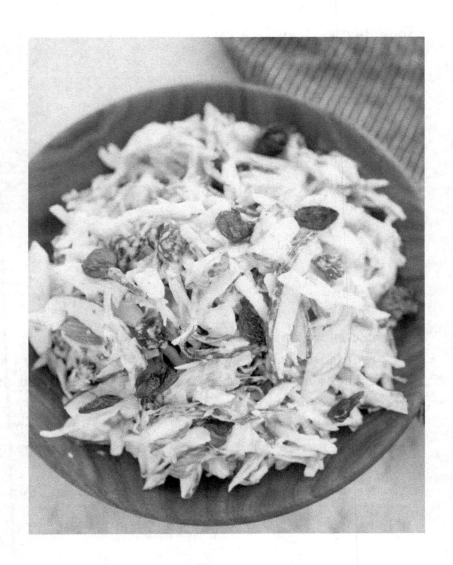

# Appetizers

## Hummus

**Ingredients** - Allergies: SF, GF, DF, EF, V, NF

1/2 cup cooked chickpeas (garbanzo beans)
1/2 small lemon
2 Tbsp. tahini
Half of a garlic clove, minced
1 tbsp. olive oil or cumin oil, plus more for serving
1/2 tsp. salt
1/4 tsp. ground cumin
2 to 3 tbsp. water
Dash of ground paprika for serving

### Instructions

Combine tahini and lemon juice and blend for 1 minute. Add the olive oil, minced garlic, cumin and the salt to tahini and lemon mixture. Process for 30 seconds, scrape sides and then process 30 seconds more.

Add half of the chickpeas to the food processor and process for 1 minute. Scrape sides, add remaining chickpeas and process for 1 to 2 minutes.

Transfer the hummus into a bowl then drizzle about 1 tbsp. of olive oil over the top and sprinkle with paprika.

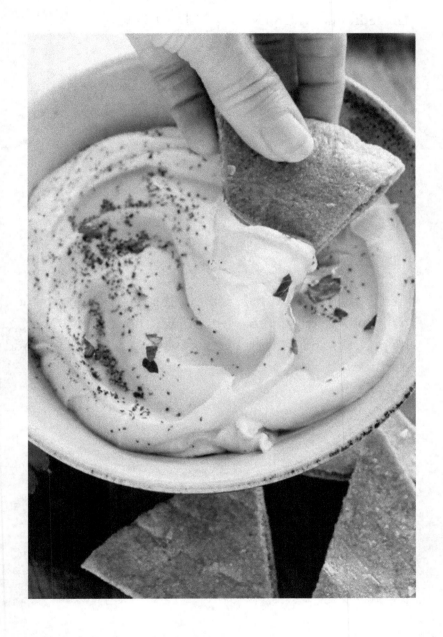

# Guacamole

**Ingredients** - Allergies: SF, GF, DF, EF, V, NF

2 ripe avocados
2 tbsp. freshly squeezed lemon juice (1 lemon)
4 dashes hot pepper sauce
1/4 cup diced onion
1 garlic clove, minced
1/2 tsp. salt
1/2 tsp. ground black pepper
1 small tomato, seeded, and small-diced

## Instructions

Cut the avocados in half, remove the pits, and scoop the flesh out. Immediately add the lemon juice, hot pepper sauce, garlic, onion, salt, and pepper and toss well. Dice avocados. Add the tomatoes. Mix well and taste for salt and pepper.

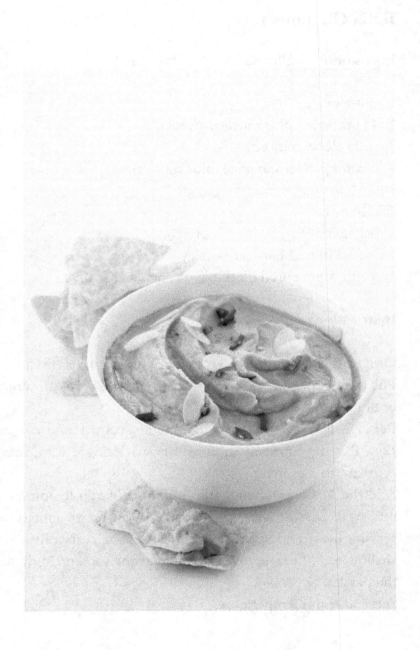

# Baba Ghanoush

**Ingredients** - Allergies: SF, GF, DF, EF, V, NF

1 eggplant
1/4 cup tahini, plus more as needed
1 garlic clove, minced
1/8 cup fresh lemon juice, plus more as needed
1 pinch ground cumin
salt, to taste
1 tbsp. extra-virgin olive oil or avocado oil
1 tbsp. chopped flat-leaf parsley
1/4 cup brine-cured black olives, such as Kalamata

## Instructions

Grill eggplant for 10 to 15 minutes. Heat the oven (375 F).
Put the eggplant to a baking sheet and bake 15-20 minutes or until very soft.
Remove from the oven, let cool, and peel off and discard the skin. Put the eggplant flesh in a bowl. Using a fork, mash the eggplant to a paste.
Add the 1/4 cup tahini, garlic, cumin, 1/4 cup lemon juice and mix well. Season with salt to taste. Transfer the mixture to a serving bowl and spread with the back of a spoon to form a shallow well. Drizzle the olive oil over the top and sprinkle with the parsley.
Serve at room temperature.

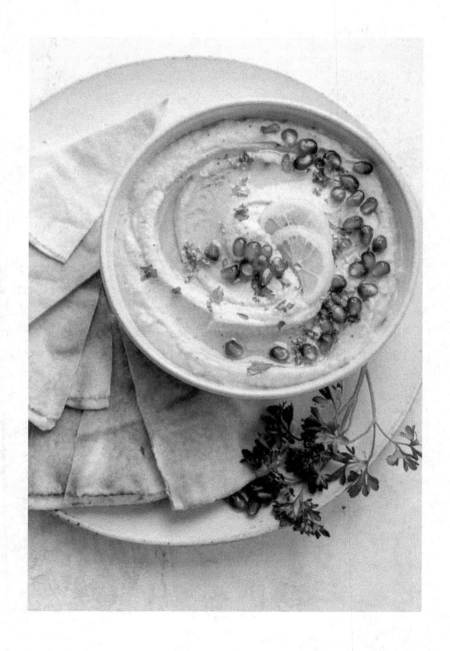

# Espinacase la Catalana

**Ingredients** - Allergies: SF, GF, DF, EF, V

1 cup spinach
1 cloves garlic
2 tbsp cashews
olive oil or avocado oil

## Instructions

Wash the spinach and trim off the stems. Steam the spinach for few minutes.
Peel and slice the garlic. Pour a few tablespoons of olive oil and cover the bottom of a frying pan. Heat pan on medium and sauté garlic for 1-2 minutes.
Add the cashews to the pan and continue to sauté for 1 minute.
Add the spinach and mix well, coating with oil. Salt to taste.

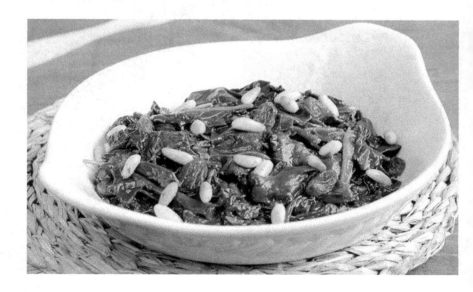

# Tapenade

**Ingredients** - Allergies: SF, GF, DF, EF, V, NF

1/4 pound olives with pit removed
2 anchovy fillets, rinsed
1 small clove garlic, minced
2 tbsp. capers
2 fresh basil leaves
1 tbsp. freshly squeezed lemon juice
1 tbsp. extra-virgin olive oil or cumin oil

## Instructions

Rinse the olives in cool water. Place all ingredients in the bowl of a food processor. Process to combine, until it becomes a coarse paste. Transfer to a bowl and serve.

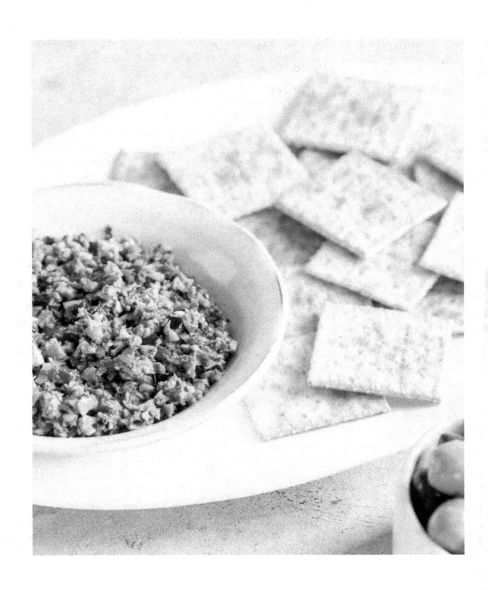

# Red Pepper Dip

**Ingredients** - Allergies: SF, GF, EF, NF

1/2 pound red peppers
1/2 cup farmers' cheese
1 Tbsp. virgin olive oil or avocado oil
1/2 tbsp minced garlic
Lemon juice, salt, basil, oregano, red pepper flakes to taste.

## Instructions

Roast the peppers. Cover them and cool for about 15 minutes. Peel the peppers and remove the seeds and stems. Chop the peppers.

Transfer the peppers and garlic to a food processor and process until smooth. Add the farmers' cheese and garlic and process until smooth.

With the machine running, add olive oil and lemon juice. Add the basil, oregano, red pepper flakes, and 1/8 tsp. salt, and process until smooth. Adjust the seasoning, to taste. Pour to a bowl and refrigerate.

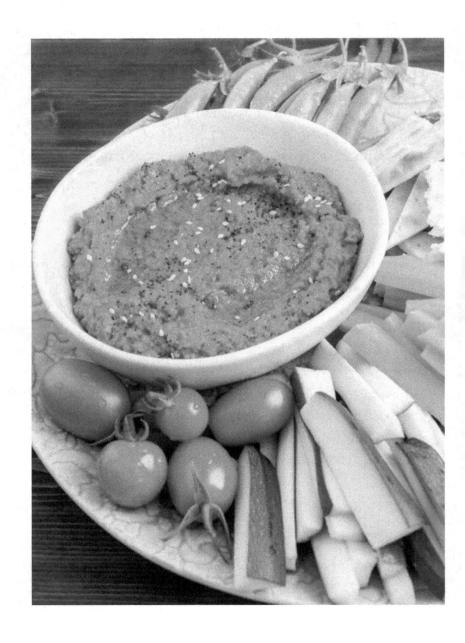

# Caponata

**Ingredients** - Allergies: SF, GF, DF

Coconut oil
1 large eggplants, cut into large chunks
1 tsp. dried oregano
Sea salt
Freshly ground black pepper
1 small onion, peeled and finely chopped
1 clove garlic, peeled and finely sliced
1 small bunch fresh flat-leaf parsley, leaves picked and stalks finely chopped
1 tbsp. salted capers, rinsed, soaked and drained
1 handful green olives, stones removed
2 tbsp. lemon juice
2 large ripe tomatoes, roughly chopped
Coconut oil
2 tbsp. slivered almonds, lightly toasted, optional

**Instructions**

Heat coconut oil in a pan and add eggplant, oregano and salt. Cook on a high heat for around 4 or 5 minutes. Add the onion, garlic and parsley stalks and continue cooking for another few minutes. Add drained capers and the olives and lemon juice. When all the juice has evaporated, add the tomatoes and simmer until tender. Season with salt and olive oil to taste before serving. Sprinkle with almonds.

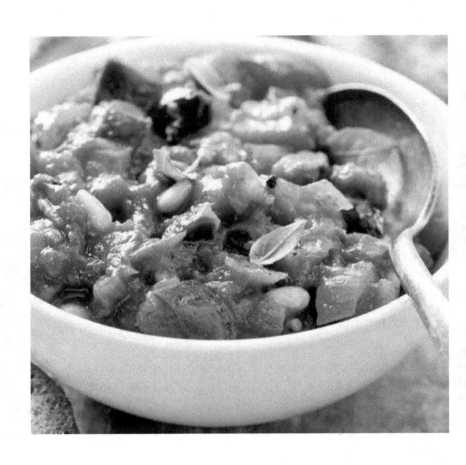

# Soups
## Cream of Broccoli Soup

**Ingredients** - Allergies: SF, GF, EF, NF

1 pound broccoli, fresh
1 cup water
1/4 tsp. salt, pepper to taste
1/4 cup tapioca flour, mixed with 1 cup cold water
1/4 cup coconut cream
1/4 cup low-fat farmers' cheese Steam or boil broccoli until it gets tender.

## Directions

Put 1 cup of water and coconut cream in top of double boiler.
Add salt, cheese and pepper. Heat until cheese gets melted.
Add broccoli. Mix water and tapioca flour in a small bowl.
Stir tapioca mixture into cheese mixture in double boiler and heat until soup thickens.

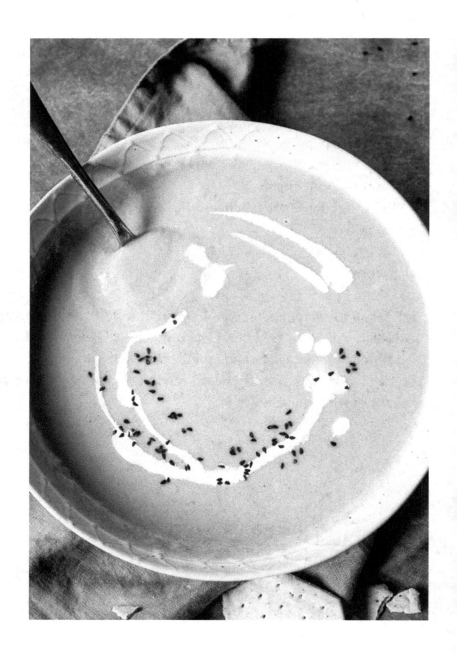

# Lentil Soup

**Ingredients** - Allergies: SF, GF, DF, EF, NF

1 tbsp. olive oil or avocado oil
1/2 cup finely chopped onion
1/4 cup chopped carrot
1/4 cup chopped celery
1 teaspoons salt
1/2 pound lentils
1/2 cup chopped tomatoes
1 quart chicken or vegetable broth
1/4 tsp. ground coriander & toasted cumin

**Instructions**

Place the olive oil into a large Dutch oven. Set over medium heat.

Once hot, add the celery, onion, carrot and salt and do until the onions are translucent. Add the lentils, tomatoes, cumin, broth and coriander and stir to combine. Increase the heat and bring just to a boil. Reduce the heat, cover and simmer at a low until the lentils are tender (approx. 35 to 40 minutes). Puree with a bender to your preferred consistency (optional).

Serve immediately.

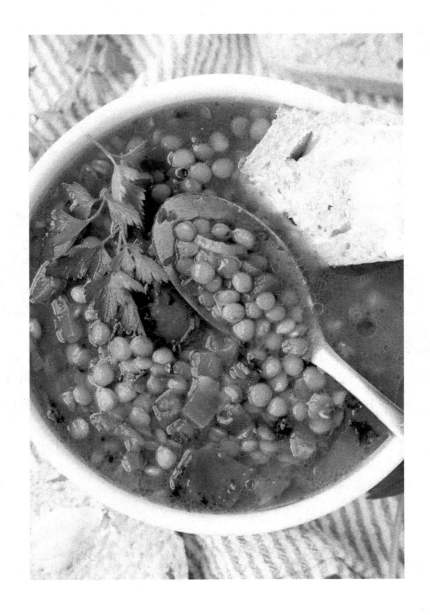

# Cold Cucumber

# Avocado Soup

**Ingredients** - Allergies: SF, GF, EF, NF

1 cucumber peeled, seeded and cut into
2-inch chunks
1 avocado, peeled
1 chopped scallions
1 cup chicken broth
1/3 cup Greek low-fat yogurt
1 tbsp. lemon juice
1/4 tsp. ground pepper, or to taste

**Garnish:**
Chopped chives, dill, mint, scallions or cucumber

**Instructions**

Combine the cucumber, avocado and scallions in a blender. Pulse until chopped.
Add yogurt, broth and lemon juice and continue until smooth.
Season with pepper and salt to taste and chill for 4 hours.
Taste for seasoning and garnish.

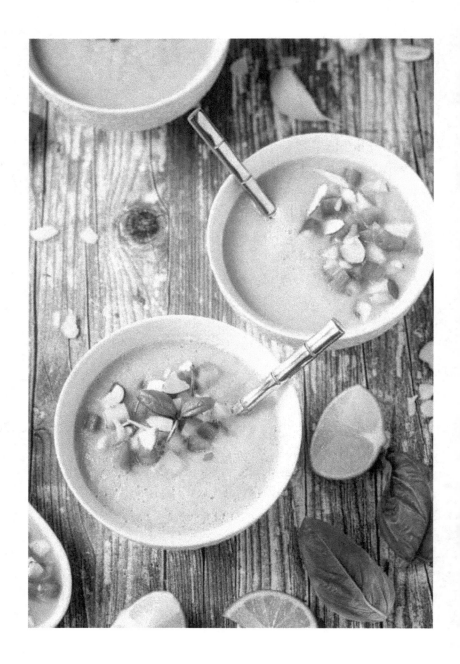

# Bouillabaisse

**Ingredients** - Allergies: SF, GF, DF, EF, NF

1 pound of 3 different kinds of fish fillets
1/4 cup Coconut oil
1 pounds of Oysters, clams, or mussels
1/3 cup cooked shrimp, crab, or lobster meat, or rock lobster tails
1/3 cup thinly sliced onions
1 Shallot or the white parts of 1 leek, thinly sliced
1 cloves garlic, crushed
1 small tomato, chopped
1/2 sweet red pepper, chopped

2 stalks celery, thinly sliced
1-inch slice of fennel or 1/2 tsp. of fennel seed
1 sprigs fresh thyme or 1/4 tsp. dried thyme
1 bay leaf
1 whole cloves
Zest of half an orange
1/4 tsp. saffron
1 teaspoons salt
1/4 tsp. ground black pepper
1/3 cup clam juice or fish broth
1 Tbps lemon juice
1/3 cup white wine

**Instructions**

In a large saucepan heat 1/8 cup of the coconut oil. When it is hot, add onions and shallots (or leeks). Sauté for a minute. Add crushed garlic, and sweet red pepper. Add celery, tomato, and fennel. Stir the vegetables until well coated. Add another 1/8 cup of coconut oil, bay leaf, thyme, cloves and the orange zest. Cook until the onion is golden. Cut fish fillets into 2-inch pieces. Add 1 cup of water and the pieces of fish to the vegetable mixture. Bring to a boil, then reduce heat and let it simmer, uncovered, for about 10 minutes. Add clams, oysters or mussels (optional) and crabmeat, shrimp or lobster tails, cut into pieces. Add salt, saffron and pepper. Add lemon juice, clam juice, and white wine. Bring to a simmer again and cook for 5 minutes longer.

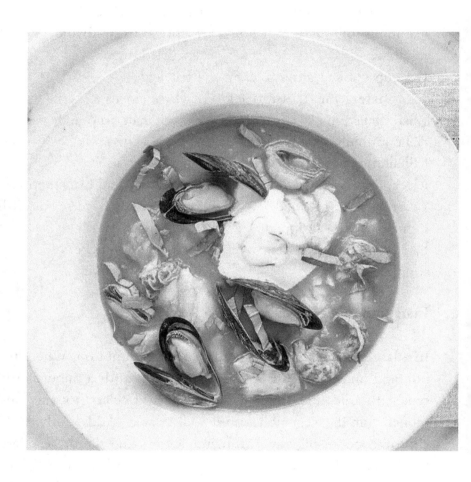

# Gaspacho

Ingredients - Allergies: SF, GF, DF, EF, V, NF

1/4 cup of flax seeds meal
1 pound tomatoes, diced
1 red pepper or 1 green pepper, diced
1 small cucumber, peeled and diced
1 cloves of garlic, peeled and crushed
1/4 cup extra virgin olive oil or cumin oil
1 tbsp. lemon juice
Salt, to taste

## Instructions

Mix the peppers, tomatoes and cucumber with the crushed garlic and olive oil in the bowl of a blender. Add flax meal to the mixture. Blend until smooth. Add salt and lemon juice to taste and stir well.
Refrigerate. Serve with black olives, hard-boiled egg, cilantro, mint or parsley.

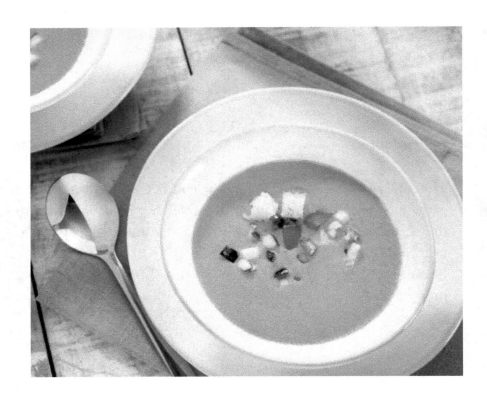

# Kale White Bean Pork Soup

**Ingredients** - Allergies: SF, GF, DF, EF, NF

1 tbsp. each extra-virgin olive oil and coconut oil
1 tbsp. chili powder
1/2 tbsp. jalapeno hot sauce
1/2 pound bone-in pork chops
Salt
2 stalks celery, chopped
1 small white onion, chopped
1 cloves garlic, chopped
1 cup chicken broth
1 cups diced tomatoes
1/2 cup cooked white beans
2 cups packed Kale

## Instructions

Preheat the broiler. Whisk hot sauce, 1 tbsp. olive oil and a pinch of chili powder in a bowl. Season the pork chops with 1/2 tsp. salt. Rub chops with the spice mixture on both sides and place them on a rack set over a baking sheet. Set aside.

Heat 1 tbsp. coconut oil in a large pot over high heat. Add the celery, garlic, onion and the remaining chili powder. Cook until onions are translucent, stirring (approx. 8 minutes).

Add tomatoes and the chicken broth to the pot. Cook and stir occasionally until reduced by about one-third (approx. 7 minutes). Add the kale and the beans.

Reduce the heat to medium, cover and cook until the kale is tender (approx. 7 minutes). Add up to 1/2 cup water if the mixture looks dry and season with salt.

In the meantime, broil the pork until browned (approx. 4 to 6 minutes). Flip and broil until cooked through. Serve with the kale and beans.

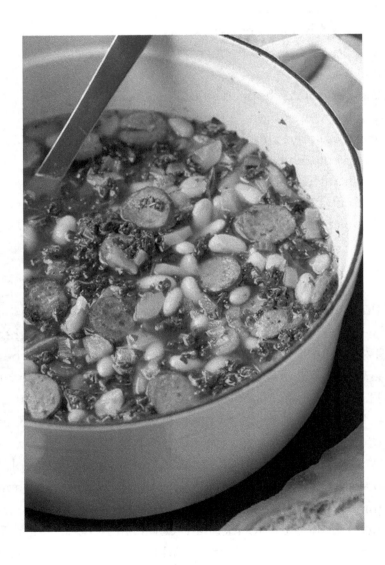

# Avgolemono – Greek lemon chicken soup

**Ingredients** - Allergies: SF, GF, DF, EF, NF

2 cups chicken broth
1/4 cup uncooked quinoa
salt and pepper
2 eggs
2 tbsp. lemon juice

## Directions

Handful fresh dill (chopped) shredded roasted chicken (optional) Bring the broth to a boil in a saucepan. Add the quinoa and cook until tender. Season with the salt and pepper. Reduce heat to low and let simmer. In a separate bowl, whisk lemon juice and the eggs until smooth. Add about 1 cup of the hot broth into the egg/lemon mixture and whisk to combine.
Add the mixture back to the saucepan. Stir until the soup becomes opaque and thickens. Add dill, salt and pepper. Optionally add chicken and serve.

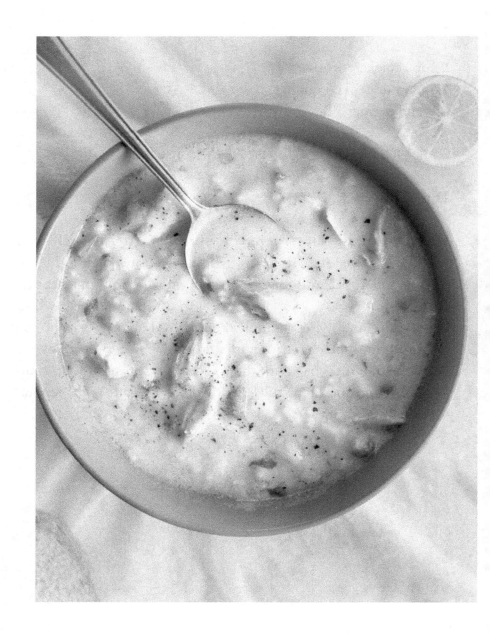

# Squash soup

**Ingredients** - Allergies: SF, GF, DF, EF, V, NF

1 small squash
1 carrot, chopped
1/2 onion (diced)
1/2 cup
coconut milk
1/4 cup water
1 tbsp. olive oil or avocado oil • Salt
Pepper
Cinnamon
Turmeric

**Instructions**

Cut the squash and spoon out the seeds. Cut it into large pieces and place on a baking sheet. Sprinkle with salt, olive oil, and pepper and bake at 375 degrees F until soft (approx. 1 hour). Let cool.
In the meantime, sauté the onions in olive oil (put it in a soup pot).
Add the carrots. Add 1/4 cup coconut milk and 1/4 cup water after few minutes and let simmer. Scoop the squash out of its skin. Add it to the soup pot. Stir to combine the ingredients and let simmer a few minutes. Add more milk or water if needed. Season to taste with the salt, pepper and spices. Blend until smooth and creamy.
Sprinkle it with toasted pumpkin seeds.

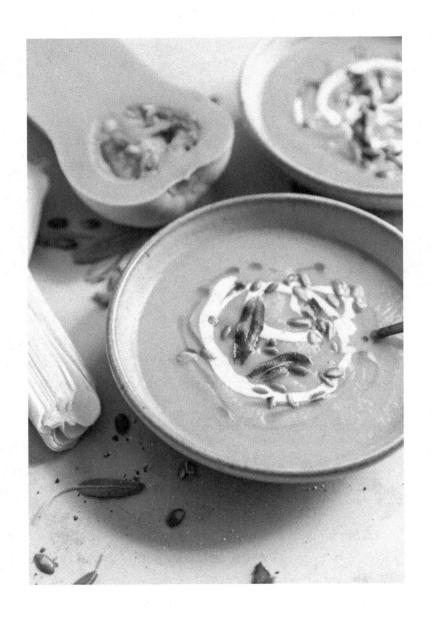

# Italian Beef Soup

**Ingredients** - Allergies: SF, GF, DF, EF, NF

1/3 pound minced beef
1 clove garlic, minced
1 cups beef broth
1 large tomato
1/2 cup sliced carrots
1/2 cup cooked beans
1 small zucchini, cubed
1 cups spinach - rinsed and torn
1/8 tsp. black pepper
1/8 tsp. salt

## Directions

Brown beef with garlic in a stockpot. Stir in broth, carrots and tomatoes. Season with salt and pepper. Reduce heat, cover, and simmer for 15 minutes.
Stir in beans with liquid and zucchini. Cover, and simmer until zucchini is tender. Remove from heat, add spinach and cover. Serve after 5 minutes.

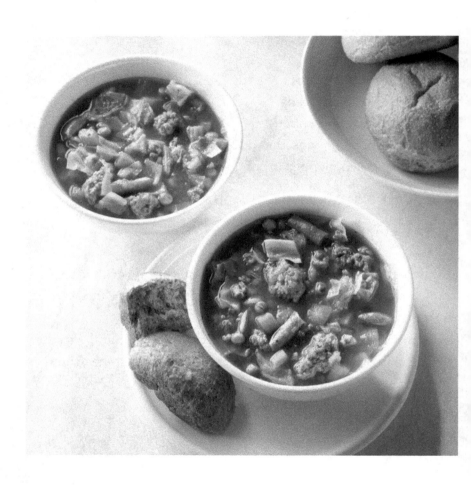

# Creamy roasted mushroom

**Ingredients** - Allergies: SF, GF, DF, EF, V, NF

1/2 pound Portobello mushrooms, cut into 1inch pieces
1/4 pound shiitake
mushrooms, stemmed
2 tbsp. olive oil or avocado oil
1 cups vegetable broth
1 tbsp. coconut oil
1/2 onion, chopped
1 garlic cloves, minced
1 tbsp. arrowroot flour
1/4 cup coconut cream
1/4 tsp. chopped thyme

## Instructions

Heat oven to 400°F. Line one large baking sheets with foil. Spread mushrooms and drizzle some olive oil on them. Season with salt and pepper and toss. Cover with foil and bake them for half an hour. Uncover and continue baking 15 minutes more. Cool slightly. Mix one half of the mushrooms with one can of broth in a blender. Set aside.
Melt coconut oil in a large pot over high heat. Add onion and garlic and sauté until onion is translucent. Add flour and stir 2 minutes. Add cream, broth, and thyme. Stir in remaining cooked mushrooms and mushroom puree. Simmer over low heat until thickened (approx. 10 minutes). Season to taste with salt and pepper.

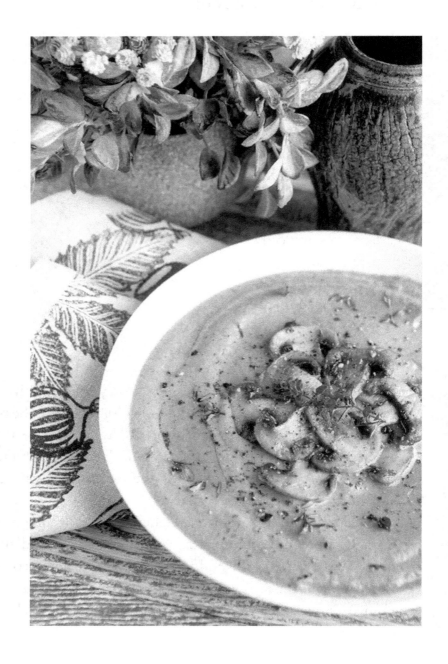

# Egg-Drop Soup

**Ingredients** - Allergies: SF, GF, DF, NF

- 2 cups quarts chicken broth
- 1 tbsps. Tapioca flour, mixed in 1/4 cup cold water
- 2 eggs, slightly beaten with a fork
- 2 scallions, chopped, including green ends

## Instructions

Bring broth to a boil. Slowly pour in the tapioca flour mixture while stirring the broth. The broth should thicken. Reduce heat and let it simmer. Mix in the eggs very slowly while stirring. As soon as the last drop of egg is in, turn off the heat. Serve with chopped scallions on top.

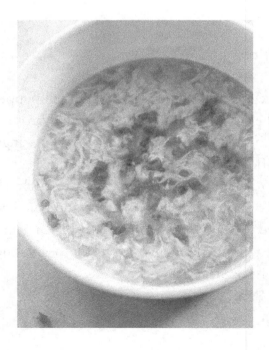

# Black Bean Soup

## Ingredients - Allergies: SF, GF, DF, EF, NF

1 Tbsp. cup Coconut Oil
1/4 cup Onion, Diced
1/4 cup Carrots, Diced
1/4 cup Green Bell Pepper, Diced
1 cup beef broth
1 pound cooked Black Beans
1 tbsp. lemon juice
1 teaspoons chopped Garlic
1 teaspoons Salt
1/4 tsp. Black Pepper, Ground
1 teaspoons Chili Powder
4 oz. pork
1 tbsp. tapioca flour
tbsp. Water

## Instructions

Place coconut oil, onion, carrot, and bell pepper in a stock pot. Cook the veggies until tender. Bring broth to a boil. Add cooked beans, broth and the remaining ingredients (except tapioca flour and 2 tbsp. water) to the vegetables. Bring that mixture to a simmer and cook approximately 15 minutes. Puree 1 quart of the soup in a blender and put back into the pot. Combine the tapioca flour and 2 tbsp. water in a separate bowl. Add the tapioca flour mixture to the bean soup and bring to a boil for 1 minute.

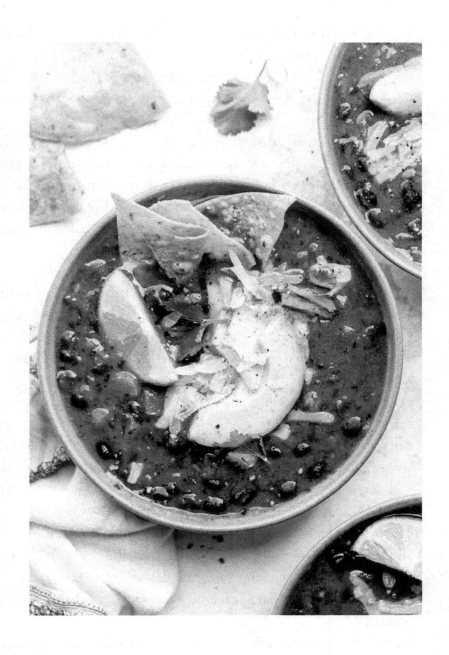

# Superfoods Smoothies

Put the liquid in first. Surrounded by tea or yogurt, the blender blades can move freely. Next, add chunks of fruits or vegetables. Leafy greens are going into the pitcher last. Preferred liquid is green tea, but you can use almond or coconut milk or herbal tea.

Start slow. If your blender has speeds, start it on low to break up big pieces of fruit. Continue blending until you get a puree. If your blender can pulse, pulse a few times before switching to a puree mode. Once you have your liquid and fruit pureed, start adding greens, very slowly. Wait until previous batch of greens has been completely blended.

Thicken? Added too much tea or coconut milk? Thicken your smoothie by adding ice cubes, flax meal, chia seeds or oatmeal. Once you get used to various tastes of smoothies, add any seaweed, spirulina, chlorella powder or ginger for additional kick. Experiment with any Superfoods in powder form at this point. Think of adding any nut butter or sesame paste too or some Superfoods oils.

Rotate! Rotate your greens; don't always drink the same smoothie! At the beginning try 2 different greens every week and later introduce third and fourth one weekly. And keep rotating them. Don't use spinach and kale all the time.

Try beets greens, they have a pinch of pink in them and that add great color to your smoothie. Here is the list of leafy green for you to try: spinach, kale, dandelion, chards, beet leaves, arugula, lettuce, collard greens, bok choy, cabbage, cilantro, parsley.

Flavor! Flavor smoothies with ground vanilla bean, cinnamon, lucuma powder, nutmeg, cloves, almond butter, cayenne pepper, ginger or just about any seeds or chopped nuts combination.

Not only are green smoothies high in nutrients, vitamins and fiber, they can also make any vegetable you probably don't like (be it kale, spinach or broccoli) taste great. The secret behind blending the perfect smoothie is using sweet fruits or nuts or seeds to give your drink a unique taste.

There's a reason kale and spinach seem to be the main ingredients in almost every green smoothie. Not only do they give smoothies their verdant color, they are also packed with calcium, protein and iron.

Although blending alone increases the accessibility of carotenoids, since the presence of fats is known to increase carotenoid absorption from leafy greens, it is possible that coconut oil, nuts and seeds in a smoothie could increase absorption further.

If you can't find some ingredient, replace it with the closest one.

CPSIA information can be obtained
at www.ICGtesting.com
Printed in the USA
BVHW090327220621
610126BV00012B/2871